I0447256

THE TRAINING PROGRAM OF LOUIS ABELE

By

CHESTER TEEGARDEN

Originally Published in 1948

PUBLISHED BY O'Faolain Patriot L L C,
Copyright 2012

info@physicalculturebooks.com

ISBN-13: 978-1475127089

ISBN-10: 1475127081

Published in the United States of America

To Order More Copies Visit:
PhysicalCultureBooks.com

FOREWORD.

These Training Programs of Louis Abele are important because they have been compiled, organized and now published so that you, the reader, may study them.

This is the culmination of my original idea. When I first became acquainted with Louis Abele I was impressed that his methods of training procedure should not be lost to humanity in general to the Muscle Culture fan in particular. Before becoming personally acquainted with Louis at the Junior National Weight Lifting Championships in St. Louis in 1939 and consequently receiving correspondence and photos from him, I had, as a quick lifting enthusiast and competitor in the AAU, been interested in the training programs of Charles Rigoulot of France. Also of Nosier of Egypt, Novak of U.S.S.R., Walker of England, Touni of Egypt, etc. Rigoulot has been for more than a score of years, the heavy weight world record holder in the two hand Clean and Jerk at 402.5 pounds. But, have Rigoulot's training schedules been recorded and published, making them available and useful to the general public ?

Objective data, unrecorded, is soon lost. Stanko and Davis have totalled more than 1,000 pounds on the 3 Olympic Lifts but have their training programs and schedules (which they did perform) become objective recorded data? Only recorded objective data are valuable to a literate people.

These Programs of Louis Abele are of value to the average reader because it acquaints him with a field of operation beyond his probably attainable horizon. But it shows you this thing has been done, therefore broadening your horizon in Muscle Culture. It is easier to follow a path than to blaze a trail. Few of us attain more than 10 per cent of our intellectual potential, so, most of us live well within •our capacity even when the energy is present and the facilities are at hand. We lack Know-How.

Abele's training can be useful to you if you adopt his system of progression in poundages and repetitions according to the ease or difficulty of performance. My advice: Study and discuss Abele.

Chester O. Teegarden

LOUIS ABELE MAKES WORLD RECORD

Philadelphia, Pennsylvania

12 February, 1940

Dear Chester:

You have my permission to use the idea which I wrote to you some time ago. If you want to write it up please refrain from writing up the Press. I have been experimenting and will have some data in the future regarding the extent of improvement that can be expected. You can mention that I will! try to have completed research on the "white mice" (the boys Louis trains) in about two months.

I am expecting to get some photos taken in New York soon. I will send some for publication in the Iron Man.

I broke the World Heavy Weight two hand snatch record in the contest at our Club (the Lighthouse Boys' Club, Philadelphia) on the tenth of February.

The former record was held by Ronald Walker of England at 292. I did 296. My total was 941. (280, 296, 365).

Yours truly,

Louis Abele

QUICK LIFTING TRAINING SCHEDULE

Dear Chester;

I was pleased to receive a letter from you so soon after the Junior Nationals. I had not expected one for some time. It seems as though you are in earnest in regard to your lifting and your desire to improve. I can not specifically advise you what to do, but I can give you my opinion regarding your problems. You wrote, in part, that you had been training for some years, three times a week. Why don't you try training six times a week? Training six times a week may make you snap out of your present slump. I have observed numerous instances of young men who have approximately the same problems as you, and they have benefited from training more often. One fellow in particular made tremendous improvement by training eight or nine times a week; once or twice in the afternoon, then every evening in the week. The extras were only partial work outs. The times between workouts enable greater effort to be utilized in each individual attempt. If I remember correctly his total jumped from 565 to 675 in four months' time as a light heavyweight. He did not work or engage in any other activity. He also slept the greater part of the day.

I tried training every day in the week and improved considerably. But as I think I told you in St. Louis, my deltoids gave out. That is, they pained me so in lifting that I had to discontinue my training. I have not come up to the lifts I made in any contest I have entered since. I had pressed 265, snatched 275, clean and jerked 340 for a total of 880.

In training every day do only presses one day and snatches or cleans the next day and presses again the third day. Do the following repetitions. I will list what I did.

Press	Snatch—all from dead hang
210 X 5	220 X 5
220 X 4	230 X 4
230 X 3	240 X 3
230 X 3	240 X 3
240 X 2	250 X 1
245 X 1	235 X 3
225 X 3	225 X 3
215 X 3	215 X 3

This is not as difficult as it looks, since you do only one lift in a workout period. Do nothing else and that means squats, dead lifts, etc. Strange as it may seem, you will more than likely improve in your squats due to the lifts. I had not squatted for about 1½ years; and when I went back to try myself, I did 15 repetitions with 400 pounds so easily that I think I could do about 20 or 22 in a couple of weeks.

It may interest you to know that Constantine Kosiras, the Greek fellow at our Club, made a remarkable improvement almost overnight. He had been doing nothing but squats for some months and then tried himself on the lifts one day. His press came up from 170 to 190, his snatch from 195 to 220, and his clean and jerk from 235 to 260. His body weight had also increased from 172 to 185, due to the squats, and previous to this new improvement in lifting.

I hope that anything I may have written will give you some helpful suggestions to incorporate in your training, and hoping I will hear from you in the near future, I remain,

Sincerely,

Louis Abele

A BIOGRAPHICAL SKETCH

29 February, 1940

This is an answer to your letter asking for a short biography of myself. I was born in the Province of Wurtemberg, Germany, on November 7, 1919. My ancestors were farmers, foresters and quarry workers. I lived in the hilly country.

We came to the United States when I was five years of age and in the following years I engaged in the ordinary activities of boyhood. I noticed early in life that I could outrun and out jump my companions with ease. I was interested in gymnastics before lifting became my greatest interest, and often remained in the gymnasium for hours. Swimming was also one of my favorite pastimes.

My first attempt to lift a bar bell resulted in my pressing one hundred pounds. I started training on progressive weight lifting and body building at the age of fifteen after watching older fellows practice lifting at the Lighthouse Boys' Club. At that time I was 5 feet 5 inches tall and weighed 130 pounds. I had an inborn desire to be stronger than the next fellow and the environment also had a good bit to do with my urge for strength. My father often spoke of our powerful ancestors and he, himself, was considered the most powerful man in the surrounding dist.

I had many teachers during my initial period of training due to the leader plan in the Lighthouse Boys' Club. When a fellow reaches 21 at the Club and is particularly suited to teach younger fellows, he is asked to stay on and become an unpaid member of the staff. His only reward is the continued use of the facilities of the Club and the pleasure of watching the progress and development of the younger members. (There are also some junior members who, because of their unusual ability in their particular activity, either sport or social, become ideal as teachers.) At present I am a junior leader. The Club has about 80 leaders.

I think I have been my own best teacher due to experimentation. The peculiar thing is that none of my experiments have failed to produce desirable results and I have, therefore, never been compelled to seek outside information. I have also learned very much from discussion with fellow lifters. We have always been receptive to any reasonable idea put forward by training1 companions even if they were much inferior in muscularity and strength. In fact, anyone who comes to our training quarters will find a heated discussion in full swing in regard to some training problem. Usually it is Kosiras and myself who are in the midst of a heated discussion.

My goal, as perhaps you are aware, is to surpass the records of Charles Rigoulot in the two hand quick lifts and Josef Manger in the two hand press. Another objective is to weigh 225 in hard muscular condition at the height of 5 feet, 9 inches. I also want to explode the theory of the dependency of muscular size on bone size. I have already done this last mentioned thing but wish really to explode it to my own satisfaction. According to the experts my 7½ inch wrist would not support any more than a 16¾ inch arm and at present my arm measures 18 inches. I hope to get it up to 19 inches.

I have always hammered away at back & leg work until I started seriously to improve my lifting, but I will make that the subject of a future letter since the multitudinous amount of leg work I have done would fill a volume.

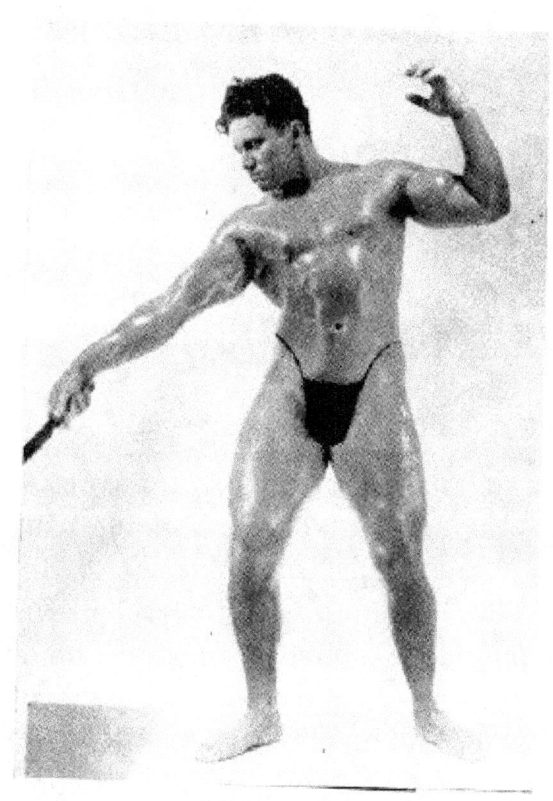

LOUIS ABELE

THE TWO ARM PRESS

18 January, 1940

Friend Chester:

Please keep this information about the Press quiet, it has not been thoroughly tested yet. Do not have any of the details made public. It has had such beneficial results on my "white mice" that I am not telling everyone.

Since you are intending to work out three times per week you should really be able to polish off some worthwhile results. Work out as follows: Start with a poundage about 35 pounds below your limit. Do one repetition. Wait five minutes and do another repetition. And so on and on until you have done twenty or more repetitions. Do this three nights per week. The second week add 2½ pounds, and so on the third and every week. When the going gets tough and you cannot finish in your specified time, about 1½ hours, cut down on your repetitions to 15 or so and rest 7 or 8 minutes between each press and finally allow yourself 10 or 12 minutes rest between each repetition when the poundage approaches your limit. Now reduce the weight 25 pounds below your limit at this time and work up again using the same procedure. When you get stuck this time take two or three weeks rest and start over again. REMEMBER, do nothing else in the line of exercises even though you get fat or if your muscles shrink a little.

MORE ABOUT THE PRESS

15 May, 1940

Friend Chester:

I believe I have some definite information now regarding the press. As I told you, practice the press every other day doing one repetition and then resting for a specified time. I explained also how I increased the weight and lengthened the time between presses. This information has been followed by several of my acquaintances, both personal and those with whom I correspond. There have been definite increases in every case over a period of several weeks. The increases as I noted in almost every instance, amounted to 15 or 20 pounds. This is strange indeed if it happens to be a coincidence that all those who tried it improved to the same extent but I would be unwilling to commit myself and say that every one will definitely improve to a similar extent. You can

add this information to the other letter
I wrote if you wish.

Yours very truly,

Louis Abele

SOME BACK WORK

14 October, 1940

I am now specializing on (back work. I have worked up to 235 X 10 consecutive dead hang snatches. I will attempt to give you my leg schedule as soon as possible.

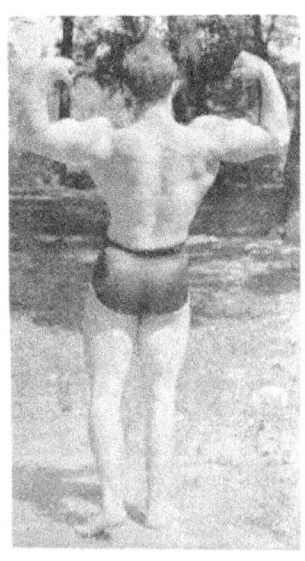

BACK POSE OF LOUIS ABELE

ABELE'S LEG PROGRAM

8 March, 1941

Friend Chester:

I was glad to hear from you again. I did not answer sooner because I have been in Cuba several weeks. Davis, Terlazzo and I gave exhibitions in Havana. I surprised myself by totalling 980: Press 310, snatch 300 and clean and jerk 370.

Regarding the leg program I have followed, I wish to make it clear that I did not reach the peak of development my legs possess at present through following a specialized leg program for two months. I did the following leg program with minor variations at three separate periods of my training each consisting of two months intensive work.

I ask you, Chester; Did you ever, during your career of lifting, see anyone whose thighs showed extreme muscular development due to such work as the proponents of the "take it easy and grow" school advise? 1 think I can answer for you; No!

You know as well as I the products of such system develop a "muscularity" that is entirely devoid of contour and woefully lacking in separation. They develop fat men's thighs and nothing more. Then when they reduce in order to bring about the transformation of smooth thighs to muscular thighs they will find to their amazement that they are practically back where they started and their gains of many inches fade away.

Do not these (take it easy and grow) gents realize it takes toil and sweat and more sweat and toil to grow muscle! To approach anything approximating some of our muscular phenomenon requires work of the most intense sort. You must literally sweat blood to get up there and let none forget it for an instant.

This tirade certainly would not do for manufacturers of exercise equipment to advocate as it would scare away all their prospects; but it, never- the less, stands as the unvarnished truth.

Let me give you an example of what I mean by intense muscle building work as followed by some one other than myself; namely, John Davis, World Heavyweight Champion. Davis, realizing his legs could stand improvement, tackled the problem and followed a squatting routine of from sixty to eighty squats in sets of over 15 each with weights above 400 pounds. The improvement in the contour and separation of his thighs has been amazing. His thighs have grown from twenty five to about twenty seven inches.

Now let me tell you of the program I followed to improve my thighs and which caused muscular tissue to grow—not fat. I started at about twenty percent below my limit. When doing the exercises I never stopped between repetitions to rest as most leg workers do. I gradually increased the poundages and stayed at the maximum repetitions.

The exercises were as follows:

1. Deep Knee Bend or Squat, twenty repetitions.

2. Leg Press, twenty repetitions.

3. Calf Exercise, twenty five repetitions. One foot at a time with toes raised on a block.

4. Step-up on a box, twenty repetitions with each leg.

5. One Leg Squat, fifteen repetitions. Note: in split position going down on forward foot to a maximum squat and balancing with the rear foot.

6. Leg Curl, fifteen repetitions.

7. Calf Exercise twenty repetitions.

8. Squat with bar bell in Jerking position, ten repetitions.

Questions by Teegarden and Abele's answers.

a. How often did you work out? Three times a week.

b. Any upper body work? No upper body work.

Followed for a two months period on three separate occasions.

Don't think I advise anyone to go at it this severely; also keep in mind to make muscles grow you must really work at it. An acquaintance of mine and incidentally one of the most muscular specimen who ever lived, (not Grimek) used to exercise so hard his joints creaked and groaned so much it was audible to a bystander. This information may be a jolt to some exercise fans, but it is, nevertheless, the truth.

Many of our best lifters work to the point of nausea time and time again when they are working near their maximum. I have worked so hard on various occasions I had to vomit. You simply do not become exceptional unless you put forth the effort. Function makes structure, by heck, and don't try fooling Nature with roundabout methods.

Cordially yours,

Louis Abele

P.S. Something I forgot to mention. I also advise the type of work Rader advises for those who approach me regarding a quick gain in bodyweight. I give them the dope straight and tell them not to expect the muscles to grow too easily because they simply won't do it.

ABELE'S BACK PROGRAM

As I explained while you visited me last (May 1942) I am a great proponent of specialization. When I first awakened to the possibilities of specialization I had been reading Mark Berry's writings in which he outlined some suggestions of previous specializers.

From my earlier experience it was possible for me to outline a program which I believe is as good as any ever evolved. I had, by this time, been steeped in the benefits of heavy leg and back work and this idea, therefore, became a basis of my program.

As is well known after a gain in bodyweight, the smaller muscle groups respond more easily to exercise than if one's bodyweight remained stable. Therefore, reason prompts me to work on the large muscle groups first, then on the smaller groups. What would be the sense of straining and striving for bigger arms and shoulders first when the leg work which causes the gain in weight and the proportion of arms to the other parts of the body produces the desired results more efficiently? It always seemed reasonable to me to bring up the legs and hips first, back and chest next, and with the consequent enlarging of the rib box and shoulder girdle, the arms, when finally called upon, will grow very easily.

Naturally, one specializes when further growth thru other methods becomes too slow. When the muscles become accustomed to a definite degree of exertion they will fail to increase in size unless they are caused to exert themselves further. This, becomes impossible after one has reached a peak in his training. If one kept increasing the work of all the muscles at one time it would not be long before rigor mortis set in. This leaves us with only one alternative: That is the specialization in one specific section of the body at one time.

As I have explained to you previously, I had done my leg program first, which lasted over a period between two and three months. I also believe I explained to you that I estimated poundages that were within my power to reach and therefore would start at a poundage that would enable me to make a gradual increase throughout the program. Any one with some measure of experience can judge how long he will continue to improve steadily and can therefore set his poundages with a fair degree of accuracy.

This is the Back Program which I followed:

> 1. Eight bent presses. Consecutive from the shoulder to overhead.

> 2. Straight leg dead lift. On a box to arches of feet.

3. Chin the bar. 10 to 12 reps, with a weight attached, usually by a rope or strap around my neck. Three variations were used: Regular and under grip and pull up to chest; over grip to chin; and behind neck.

4. Stationary rowing exercise. 12 repetitions.

5. One arm rowing with a kettle bell. 15 repetitions,

6. Two arm snatch. 10 consecutive times, no pause, from dead hang.

7. Two hand clean in the same manner as the snatch but later eliminated because it was too tough.

8. Regular dead lift. 10 to 12 repetitions.

When I used to do snatches and cleans I had to pry my fingers off the bar and often would tear callouses off. It also caused such violent breathing my teeth ached.

During a specialized program on any part of the body the unused parts of the anatomy will naturally lose some shape and tone. But do not lose sight of your principle aim. After these periods of specialization are over the unused parts will snap back to their original size and shape in two weeks time.

These are some of my best measurements and lifts which you requested. Press 315. Snatch 310. Clean 375 (no jerk). Jerk 375 (no clean). Bent Press 225 at 185 pounds bodyweight. Best Deep Knee Bends: 400 X 18, 450 X 10, 475 X 7.

Neck 18. Arms 18½. Chest 49. Forearms 14. Wrists 7.5, Waist 36. Hips 43. Thighs 28.5. Calf 17.5 Ankles 9%. Height 5'9". Age 21. Weight when dressed, 238,

Yours truly,

Louis Abele